YOUR KNOWLEDGE HAS VALUE

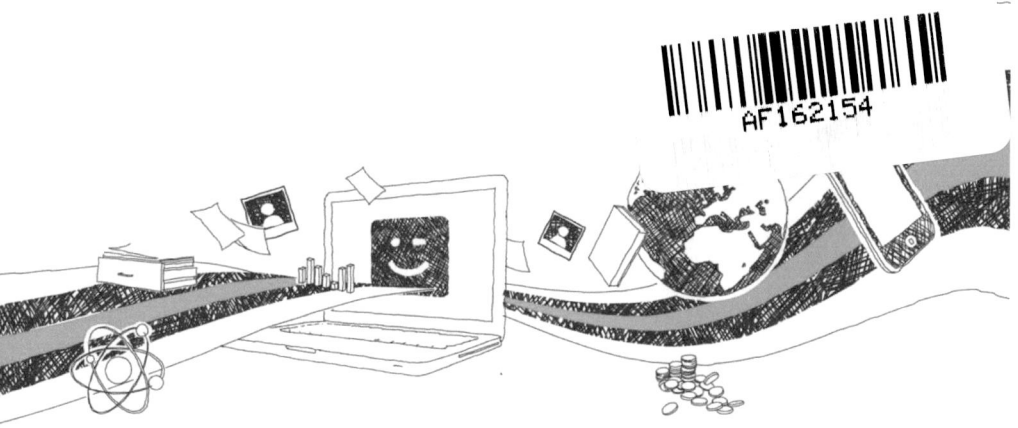

- We will publish your bachelor's and
  master's thesis, essays and papers

- Your own eBook and book -
  sold worldwide in all relevant shops

- Earn money with each sale

Upload your text at www.GRIN.com
and publish for free

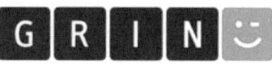

Bibliographic information published by the German National Library:

The German National Library lists this publication in the National Bibliography; detailed bibliographic data are available on the Internet at http://dnb.dnb.de .

This book is copyright material and must not be copied, reproduced, transferred, distributed, leased, licensed or publicly performed or used in any way except as specifically permitted in writing by the publishers, as allowed under the terms and conditions under which it was purchased or as strictly permitted by applicable copyright law. Any unauthorized distribution or use of this text may be a direct infringement of the author s and publisher s rights and those responsible may be liable in law accordingly.

Imprint:

Copyright © 2017 GRIN Verlag, Open Publishing GmbH
Print and binding: Books on Demand GmbH, Norderstedt Germany
ISBN: 9783668582323

This book at GRIN:

http://www.grin.com/en/e-book/381247/the-differences-between-postmortem-and-antemortem-injuries

Patrick Kimuyu

The differences between postmortem and antemortem injuries

GRIN Publishing

GRIN - Your knowledge has value

Since its foundation in 1998, GRIN has specialized in publishing academic texts by students, college teachers and other academics as e-book and printed book. The website www.grin.com is an ideal platform for presenting term papers, final papers, scientific essays, dissertations and specialist books.

Visit us on the internet:

http://www.grin.com/

http://www.facebook.com/grincom

http://www.twitter.com/grin_com

Introduction

Autopsy is a valuable procedure performed by a qualified physician to assess the quality of patient care to evaluate clinical diagnostic accuracy. In addition, autopsy determines the effectiveness and impact of therapeutic regimens in discovering and defining new or changing diseases to increase the understanding of biological processes of disease. It also helps in augmenting clinical and basic research, to provide accurate public health and education as it relates to disease and medico - legal factual information. The benefits of forensic autopsy in criminology are undisputed; it allows the pathologist to see, and describe findings that were previously demonstrated and confirmed through the use of histology for confirmation (Dolinak, Lew & Matshes 2005).

In practice, there is abundant evidence that clinical diagnosis still have room for improvement and that autopsy has much to contribute to the improvement of patient care. However, forensic pathology requires extensive understanding on post-mortem and ante-mortem differences for accurate reporting of post-mortem examinations. Therefore, this paper will provide comparisons between ante-mortem and post-mortem injuries. It will also attempt to demystify the criticism surrounding autopsy (post-mortem) by evaluating the drawbacks associated to all the methods applied in the assessment of bruises.

Ante-mortem and Post-mortem

Post-mortem refers to a forensic investigation of the cause of death, and it is done after the occurrence of the death. Ideally, post-mortem examination results are based on the form of injuries detected. In practice, there are two types of injuries involved in forensic pathology; ante-mortem injuries and post-mortem injuries. Ante-mortem injuries occur before death whereas post-mortem injuries occur after death. Therefore, ante-mortem refers to events occurring prior to death.

Comparison of Ante-mortem and Post-mortem Injuries

Ordinarily, the nature of injuries is used as the principal factor for differentiating ante-mortem injuries from post-mortem injuries. Therefore, comparison between ante-mortem and post-mortem injuries can be established with the use of the appearances of the bruise or wound.

In ante-mortem injuries, haemorrhage is associated with clotting in which clots are laminated, firm and variegated (Greaves 2000). Haemorrhage is characterized with copious amounts from arterial vessels (Bardale 2011). Post-mortem slight haemorrhage occurs on the venous vessels in which clots are absent, or they are soft, non-laminated with friable chicken-fat (yellow) appearance (Vanezis 2001).

In addition, ante-mortem wound edges appear gaped, averted and swollen whereas post-mortem wound edges are apposed without swellings.

On the other hand, the interpretation of bruises serves as a principal approach for the differentiation of ante-mortem and post-mortem injuries. Ordinarily, the appearance of bruises is indicative of the cause and time when the bruise occurred. However, it is worth noting that the location of the bruise is considered quite useful in forensic examinations. Some body parts are more likely to sustain bruises than others. For instance, bruises are known to occur more readily where there is a loose tissue such as eyebrows or subcutaneous fat than in areas where a tissue is strongly supported. In addition, the nature of the surface and force involved determines the intensity, shape, pattern and the size of the resultant bruise (Vanezis 2001). Therefore, it is quite easy to determine the nature of object used in causing the injury although there are other factors for consideration.

In general, ante-mortem bruises can be differentiated from post-mortem bruises by the use of the principal characteristics observed in histological aging. Ideally, histological ageing is used in dating ante-mortem bruises. Bruises undergo histological changes from the date of occurrence to healing. Shortly after the occurrence of a bruise, inflammation occurs in which haemostatic and vascular response occurs. This takes place within one to three days after injury. The second phase includes the regeneration of connective and epithelial tissues which occurs up to 14 days whereas scar formation results after several months (Vanezis 2001). Therefore, these changes aid in differentiating ante-mortem from post-mortem bruises. In practice, ante-mortem bruises manifest any of these characteristics, but post-mortem bruises do not show all these features because dead cells do not undergo such biological processes.

Assessment Methods

Some of the most reliable methods applied in distinguishing ante-mortem from post-mortem injuries include enzyme histochemistry, microscopy and serology. Other methods used in the assessment of bruises are direct gross examination of the dead body, objective colour assessment and gross naked eye and photographic assessment.

Enzyme histochemistry involves the quantification of various enzymes in the body to determine the time when the bruise occurred. Ordinarily, enzyme histochemistry for ante-mortem injuries shows positive and negative vital reactions. In contrast, vital reactions are absent in post-mortem injuries (Bardale 2011). Another significant biochemical diagnostic approach for distinguishing ante-mortem from post-mortem injuries is the quantification of Leukotriene B4 (LTB4) with HPLC. In practice, Leukotriene B4 is present in ante-mortem injuries, but it is absent in post-mortem injuries (He & Zhu 1996).

Despite the benefits related to biochemical assessment of injuries, it encompasses several drawbacks. For instance, decomposition of the body causes degradation of some of the most reliable enzymes contained in haemoglobin and this may lead to misinterpretation of the bruise (Vanezis 2001). In addition, serotonin and histamine which are the principal components assayed during biochemical assessment degrade upon the putrefaction of the victim's body.

On the other hand, microscopy for ante-mortem injuries show RBC and leukocyte infiltration within muscle fibres in which platelets are present. In post-mortem injuries, microscopy does not show RBC infiltration or platelets presence in clots, and serology does not indicate an increase of histamine and serotonin content (Waters 2010).

In most cases, microscopic examination is based on determining the presence of haemosiderin in the body. Ordinarily, haemosiderin is produced in the body, shortly after death. However, haemosiderin deposits appear in different body organs in variable time intervals (Akgoz, Eren, Fedakar & Turkmen 2008). For instance, haemosiderin occurs in subcutaneous tissue in 24-48 hours after injury while its appearance in the brain takes 4 days (Vanezis 2001).

Therefore, this temporal differences compromise the accuracy of microscopic assessment; thus, presenting difficulties in differentiating ante-mortem injuries from post-mortem injuries.

Conclusion

In a brief conclusion, the value of autopsy (post-mortem) is immense in improving patient care despite the criticism from physicians. However, an extensive understanding on ante-mortem and post-mortem injuries is required for accurate pathological reporting. Currently, there are different methods for distinguishing ante-mortem from post-mortem injuries although the quantification of Leukotriene B_4 appears the most reliable approach. Unfortunately, this technique has not yet been adopted in forensic medicine for biochemical assessment of bruises.

Despite the significance of autopsy, criticism has always compromised its application because all assessment methods encompass numerous drawbacks (Joseph 2001). Therefore, post-mortem examination should involve several methods to address the challenge of misinterpretation when a single method is applied.

References

Akgoz, S, Eren, B, Fedakar, R & Turkmen, N 2008, The Significance of Haemosiderin Deposition in the Lungs and Organs of the Mononucleated Macrophage Resorption System in Infants and Children, *J Korean Med Sci.*, vol. 23(6): Pp. 1020–1026. 10.3346/jkms.2008.23.6.1020

Bardale, R 2011, *Principles of forensic medicine and toxicology*, London, UK: JP Medical Ltd.

Dolinak, D. Lew, E & Matshes, E 2005, *Forensic pathology: principles and practice*. Waltham, MA: Academic Press.

Greaves, M 2000, *Haemorrhage, haemostasis and thrombosis. In:*

He, L. & Zhu, J 1996, Distinguishing ante-mortem from post-mortem injuries by LTB, quantification, *Forensic Science International*, vol. 81, Pp. 11-16.

Joseph, S 2001, The pathology of trauma. *Archives of Pathology & Laboratory Medicine*, vol. 125(12), Pp. 1616.

London, UK: Arnold.

Mason JK, Purdue BN, eds. Pathology of trauma, 3rd ed.

Vanezis, P 2001, Interpreting bruises at necropsy, *J Clin Pathol.*, vol. 54, Pp. 348–355.

Waters, B 2010, *Handbook of autopsy practice,* New York, NY: Springer.

The Significance of Hemosiderin Deposition in the Lungs and Organs of the Mononucleated Macrophage Resorption System in Infants and Children

YOUR KNOWLEDGE HAS VALUE

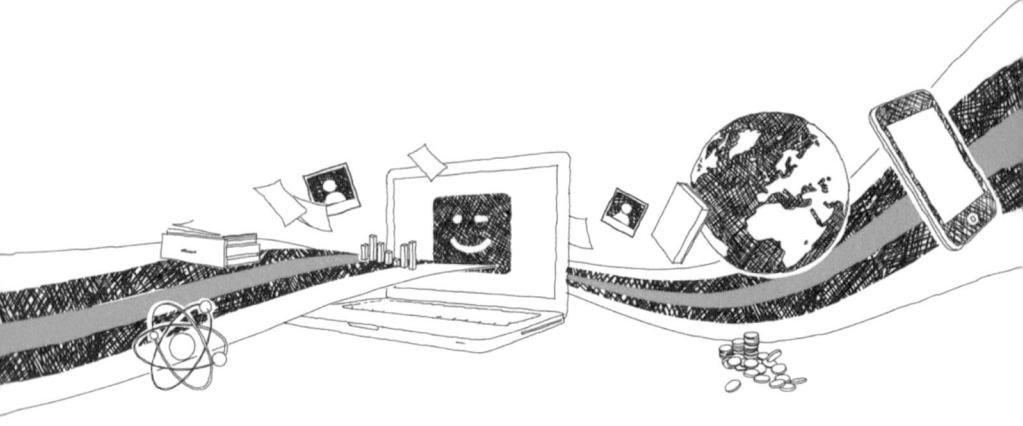

- We will publish your bachelor's and master's thesis, essays and papers

- Your own eBook and book - sold worldwide in all relevant shops

- Earn money with each sale

Upload your text at www.GRIN.com
and publish for free

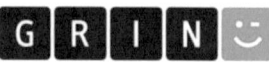